Copyright 2023

All right reserved.No part of this book should be reproduced without express permission of the author.

Reproduction of all or any part of this book is punishable unders relevant law.

Table of Contents

PREVIEW 4

HERPES DIET RECIPES 5

BREAKFAST 5

1. Overnight Merguez and Mushroom Strata 5

2. Hammy Breakfast Hotdish.. 9

3. Double Chocolate Croissant French Toast Casserole 13

4. Shannon Sarna's Basic Challah 16

5. Bubble Sweet Waffles... 19

6. Breakfast Tacos! 22

7. Mexican Breakfast Bowls... 24

8. Succotash with Poached Eggs and Herb Oil 26

9. Creamy Polenta with Eggs, Chorizo and Cilantro 29

10. Herby Smashed Potatoes 32

LUNCH.. 35

11. Tender, Golden Venezulean Corn Pancakes................ 35

12. Caprese Sandwich.. 38

13. Homemade Bread Is Made with Ground Sausage Rolled in Pizza Dough 40

14. Lentil Bolognese 44

15. Classic Deli Turkey Salad Tossed in A Mayo-Based 47

16. Moroccan Lentil and Chickpea Soup 49

17. Dijon Mustard and Tangy Sauerkraut................. 52

18. Navy Bean Soup.............................. 54

19. Soba Noodle Salad............................ 57

20. Creamy Broccoli Soup with Pesto.................. 59

DINNER 62

21. Pan-Roasted Chicken with Grapes................. 62

22. Cheesy-Filled Pasta Even Cheesier 65

23. Classic with Loads Of Bacon 68

24.Baked Chicken Shawarma (Vegan Adaptable!) 71

25. Croque Monsieur................................ 74

26. Savory Mushroom Crepes with Spaghetti Squash and Sage........ 77

27. Classic Italian Dish 82

28. Zucchini, Corn and Basil Stir-Fry with Tofu, Shrimp or Chicken ... 85

29. Cottage Pie 87

30. Vegan Tacos with Smoky Chipotle Portobellos 93

Herpes simplex virus type 1 (HSV-1) causes oral herpes, which usually affects the mouth and surrounding skin but can also affect the genital region.

herpes simplex virus type 2 (HSV-2) typically causes genital herpes, usually sexually transmitted.

There is no cure for herpes, but treatment can help manage symptoms and reduce the likelihood of outbreaks recurring and transmission to partners.

HSV is a common virus. According to the World Health Organization (WHO) Trusted Source, around 67% of people under age 50 globally have an HSV-1 infection, and 13% under age 50 have an HSV-2 infection.

In this article, we describe the symptoms of genital and oral herpes, how to treat them, and how to prevent these infections.

BREAKFAST

1. Overnight Merguez and Mushroom Strata

Prep Time: 30 Minutes

Cook Time: 1Hour 10 Minutes

Yield: serves 8 - 10

Ingredients

- 2 tablespoons salted or unsalted butter
- 1 (16- to 18-ounce) loaf unsliced levain or sourdough bread
- 1 small or 1/2 medium yellow onion
- 3 cloves garlic
- 8 ounces cremini mushrooms
- 4 medium scallions
- 8 ounces Gruyère cheese
- 12 ounces uncooked merguez sausage

- 1 tablespoon olive oil, plus more as needed
- 1 1/2 teaspoons salt, divided
- 1 teaspoon freshly ground black pepper, divided
- 8 large eggs
- 1 1/2 cups whole milk
- 1 cup heavy cream
- 2 tablespoons harissa sauce, such as Mina

Instructions

1. Let 2 tablespoons salted or unsalted butter sit at room temperature until softened.
2. Meanwhile, if you are using fresh bread, arrange a rack in the middle of the oven and heat the oven to 250°F (skip this toasting step if you are using fresh bread and just cut or tear it). Cut or tear 1 (16- to 18-ounce) loaf levain bread into rough 1-inch pieces (10 to 12 cups). Place in an even layer on a rimmed baking sheet. Bake until just starting to dry out but not browned, about 10 minutes. Set aside to cool.
3. Coat a 9x13-inch baking dish with half of softened butter, then coat a sheet of aluminum foil with the remaining butter.

4. Dice 1 small or 1/2 medium yellow onion (about 3/4 cup) and finely chop 3 garlic cloves. Trim and cut 8 ounces cremini mushrooms about 1/2-inch thick (about 2 cups). Thinly slice 4 medium scallions (about 1/2 cup). Grate 8 ounces Gruyère cheese on the large holes of a box grater (about 2 cups). Remove the casings from 12 ounces merguez sausage.

5. Heat 1 tablespoon olive oil in a large skillet over medium heat until shimmering. Add the sausage, use a wooden spoon to break it up into bite-sized pieces, and cook until cooked through and browned, 4 to 7 minutes.

6. Transfer the sausage with a slotted spoon to a large bowl. Remove all but 2 tablespoons of grease from the pan. (If there is less than 2 tablespoons grease, make up the difference with olive oil.) Add the onion and garlic to the skillet and cook over medium heat, stirring occasionally, until the onion is starting to soften, about 3 minutes.

7. Add the mushrooms, season with 1/2 teaspoon of the kosher salt and 1/2 teaspoon of the black pepper, and increase the heat to medium-high. Cook, stirring occasionally, until the liquid the mushrooms release is mostly evaporated and they begin to brown, 6 to 8

minutes. Meanwhile, place 8 large eggs, 1 1/2 cups whole milk, 1 cup heavy cream, 2 tablespoons harissa sauce, the remaining 1 teaspoon kosher salt, and remaining 1/2 teaspoon black pepper in a large bowl and whisk to combine.

8. When the mushrooms are ready, transfer to the bowl with the sausage. Add the bread, half of the cheese, and half of the scallions, and toss to combine. Transfer to the baking dish and spread into an even layer. Pour the milk mixture evenly over everything, then sprinkle with the remaining cheese. Cover the baking dish tightly with the foil butter-side down and refrigerate for at least 1 hour or up to 24 hours. Cover and refrigerate the remaining scallions.

9. Arrange a rack in the middle of the oven and heat the oven to 375°F. Let the strata sit at room temperature while the oven heats.

10. Bake covered for 30 minutes. Uncover and bake until the eggs are set, the top is browned, and the edges are crispy, about 20 minutes more. Sprinkle the reserved scallions on top and let cool for 10 minutes before serving.

2. Hammy Breakfast Hotdish

Prep Time: 30 Minutes

Cook Time: 1 Hour 10 Minutes

Yield: serves 8-10

Ingredients

- 1 medium yellow onion
- 3 medium leeks (to get 2 loosely packed cups 1/2-inch-wide leek strips)
- 12 ounces ham steak, or 2 1/2 cups diced cooked ham
- 1 large clove garlic
- 1/2 bunch asparagus (8 ounces)
- 2 tablespoons olive oil, divided
- 1 3/4 teaspoons salt, divided
- 1/2 teaspoon freshly ground black pepper, divided, plus more as needed
- 1 cup frozen peas
- 6 to 7 ounces sharp white cheddar cheese
- 8 large eggs
- 1 1/2 cups heavy cream
- 1 tablespoon Dijon mustard

- 4 ounces cream cheese

- 22 to 28 ounces frozen potato tots

- 2 tablespoons chopped fresh dill or chopped fresh chives, and hot sauce, for serving

Instructions

1. Arrange a rack in the upper third of the oven and heat the oven to 350°F.

2. Finely chop 1 medium yellow onion (1 1/2 cups) and place in a medium bowl. Halve the white and light green parts of 3 medium leeks lengthwise, then cut crosswise into 1/2-inch-thick strips until you have 2 cups. Rinse well, drain, and add to the bowl of onion.

3. Dice 12 ounces ham steak (about 2 1/2 cups). Mince 1 large garlic clove. Trim and cut 1/2 bunch asparagus crosswise into 1-inch pieces (2 cups).

4. Heat 1 tablespoon of the olive oil in a 3- to 4-quart braiser over medium-high heat until shimmering (or cook in a large frying pan and bake in a greased 9x13-inch baking dish). Add the ham and cook until golden-brown, 4 to 5 minutes.

5. Add the remaining 1 tablespoon olive oil, onion, and leeks to the pan. Season with 1 teaspoon of the kosher

salt and 1/4 teaspoon black pepper. Cook until translucent and fragrant, 4 to 5 minutes. (You want the veggies to be cooked three-quarters of the way, because they will continue to cook in the oven.)

6. Add the asparagus and garlic and sauté until just tender, about 4 minutes. (There shouldn't be too much color on the vegetables.)

7. Add 1 cup frozen peas. Stir to combine, then remove from the heat. Let cool slightly while you make the custard filling. (If using a 9x13-inch baking dish, transfer to the dish and spread into an even layer.) Meanwhile, grate 6 to 7 ounces sharp white cheddar cheese on the large holes of a box grater (about 1 3/4 cups).

8. Place 8 large eggs, 1 1/2 cups heavy cream, 1 tablespoon Dijon mustard, 1/2 teaspoon of the kosher salt, and a few grinds of black pepper in a large bowl and whisk to combine. Pour over the veggie and ham mixture. (The vegetables should be visible and not swimming in the eggy mixture. That way the potato tots don't sink!)

9. Cut 4 ounces cream cheese into 12 pieces and scatter over the vegetable-and-egg mixture. Sprinkle evenly with the cheddar.

10. Arrange 22 to 28 ounces frozen potato tots side-by-side in a uniform pattern on top of the custard filling. Sprinkle with the remaining 1/4 teaspoon kosher salt and 1/4 teaspoon black pepper. (If you have remaining tots, bake them off and snack on them later!)

11. Bake until the potato tots are golden-brown and the egg mixture is set, 40 to 55 minutes. (A thin knife inserted into the center should come out clean.) Meanwhile, finely chop until you have 2 tablespoons fresh dill or fresh chives.

12. Sprinkle with the dill or chives, and a few splashes of hot sauce before serving.

3. Double Chocolate Croissant French Toast Casserole

Prep Time: 30 Minutes

Cook Time: 50 Minutes

Yield: serves 8

Ingredients

Cooking spray

- 4 to 6 stale large croissants (10 to 12 ounces total)
- 1 (10-ounce) bag mini chocolate chips (about 1 1/2 cups), divided
- 6 large eggs
- 2 cups chocolate milk
- 1 cup heavy cream
- 3 tablespoons packed light or dark brown sugar (optional)
- 1 teaspoon vanilla extract
- 1 teaspoon ground cinnamon
- 1/2 teaspoon salt
- Whipped cream and maple syrup, for serving

Instructions

1. Lightly coat a 9x13-inch baking dish with cooking spray.

2. Halve 4 to 6 stale large croissants lengthwise and place them in the prepared pan, overlapping them as needed but as little as possible to fill the pan completely. Sprinkle 1 cup of the mini chocolate chips in between the slices.

3. Place 6 large eggs in a large bowl and whisk until light and foamy. Add 2 cups chocolate milk, 1 cup heavy cream, 3 tablespoons packed brown sugar if desired, 1 teaspoon vanilla extract, 1 teaspoon ground cinnamon, and 1/2 teaspoon kosher salt, and whisk until combined.

4. Slowly pour the mixture over the croissants, giving each individual slice a few seconds to absorb as much of the liquid as it can. Use the back of a spoon to press gently on the croissants to help them absorb the liquid. Cover the baking dish and refrigerate at least 4 hours but preferably overnight.

5. Arrange a rack in the middle of the oven and heat the oven to 350°F.

6. Uncover the baking dish. Sprinkle the remaining mini chocolate chips (about 1/2 cup) evenly over the

croissants. Bake until crispy and golden-brown, puffed around the edges, and a tester inserted in the middle comes out clean, 50 to 55 minutes. Let cool for 5 minutes before serving with whipped cream and maple syrup.

4. Shannon Sarna's Basic Challah

Prep Time: 30 Minutes

Cook Time: 24 Minutes

Yield: serves 8

Ingredients

- 1 1/4 cups lukewarm water (100°F to 110°F)
- 2 (1/4-ounce) packets active dry or instant yeast (4 1/2 teaspoons)
- 3/4 cup plus 1/2 teaspoon granulated sugar, divided
- 5 cups bread flour, preferably King Arthur, divided, plus more for dusting
- 2 1/2 teaspoons salt
- 1/4 cup vegetable oil, plus more for the bowl
- 3 large eggs, divided
- 2 to 4 tablespoons sesame seeds, poppy seeds, nigella seeds, flaky or coarse salt, or everything bagel seasoning (optional)

Instructions

Make the dough:

1. Place 1 1/4 cups lukewarm water in a small bowl. Sprinkle with 2 packets active dry or instant yeast and 1/2 teaspoon of the granulated sugar, and stir to combine. Let sit until foamy on top, about 5 minutes. If it doesn't smelly "yeasty" or bubble up, throw it out and start again with new yeast. Meanwhile, place 1 1/2 cups of the bread flour, the remaining 3/4 cup granulated sugar, and 2 1/2 teaspoons kosher salt in the bowl of a stand mixer.

2. When the yeast is ready, mix the flour mixture with the whisk attachment on medium speed until combined, 1 to 2 minutes. Add the water-yeast mixture and 1/4 cup vegetable oil and mix on high speed until smooth, about 3 minutes.

3. Stop the mixer and switch to the dough hook attachment. Add the remaining 3 1/2 cups bread flour and 2 of the large eggs. Mix on high speed until the dough is smooth and pulling away from the sides of the bowl, about 5 minutes.

4. Lightly coat a large bowl with vegetable oil and transfer the dough into the bowl. Cover the bowl with a damp kitchen towel or plastic wrap. Let rise in a

warm place until doubled in bulk and puffy, about 3 hours at room temperature, or overnight in the refrigerator.

5. Assemble and bake:

6. If the dough has been refrigerated, let it sit at room temperature for 1 hour. Line a baking sheet with parchment paper or a silicone baking mat.

7. Transfer the dough onto a very lightly floured work surface. Divide into two portions (about 22 ounces each). Braid each portion into the desired shape. Transfer to the baking sheet, spacing them evenly apart. Let the challah rise uncovered until risen by about 1/2 inch and puffed, 25 to 35 minutes. This step is very important to ensure a light and fluffy challah.

8. Meanwhile, arrange a rack in the middle of the oven and heat the oven to 375°F. Place the remaining 1 large egg in a small bowl and beat with a fork to break up.

9. Brush the egg wash liberally over the challah. Sprinkle each loaf with 1 to 2 tablespoons of topping if desired.

10. Bake until the challah is golden on the outside and sounds hollow when you "knock" on the bottom, 24 to 28 minutes. Transfer to a wire rack and let cool completely before serving or freezing.

5. Bubble Sweet Waffles

Prep Time: 30 Minutes

Cook Time: 24 Minutes

Yield: serves 8

Ingredients

- 1 1/2 cups all-purpose flour
- 3/4 cup granulated sugar
- 2 teaspoons cornstarch
- 2 teaspoons baking powder
- 1/2 teaspoon kosher salt
- 2 large eggs
- 1/2 cup milk
- 1/2 cup water
- 3 tablespoons canola or vegetable oil
- 1 teaspoon vanilla extract
- Nonstick cooking spray

For serving (optional):

- Whipped cream
- Ice cream

- Sliced strawberries

- Fresh raspberries or blueberries

- Powdered sugar

- Nutella

- Chocolate sauce

Instructions

1. Arrange a rack in the middle of the oven and heat the oven to 200°F.

2. Place 1 1/2 cups all-purpose flour, 3/4 cup granulated sugar, 2 teaspoons cornstarch, 2 teaspoons baking powder, and 1/2 teaspoon kosher salt in a large bowl and whisk to combine. If you have one, use a spouted bowl.

3. Lightly beat 2 large eggs in a medium bowl. Add 1/2 cup milk, 1/2 cup water, 3 tablespoons canola or vegetable oil, and 1 teaspoon vanilla extract, and whisk to combine. Pour into the flour mixture and whisk until smooth and no streaks of flour remain.

4. Heat the bubble waffle maker according to the manufacturer instructions. Spray both sides of the waffle maker with cooking spray.

5. If not using a spouted bowl, transfer the batter to a large, spouted measuring cup. Pour the batter into the waffle maker, filling each well all the way. Do not worry so much about the space between the wells; if you try to cover the whole surface, you will overfill the waffle maker. Cook according to the manufacturer's instructions, or for 2 minutes, then flip the waffle maker over and cook until golden-brown all over, 2 minutes more. Do not open the waffle maker until the cook time is up. (You will need 2/3 to 3/4 cup batter per waffle. Consult the manufacturer's instructions for each model for specific guidelines.)

6. Transfer cooked waffles to a baking sheet and keep warm in the oven. If you plan to fold and fill the bubble waffle, drape over a rolling pin or glass immediately after it comes out of the waffle maker, when it is soft and easily pliable. The waffle will firm up as it cools.

6. Breakfast Tacos!

Prep Time: 30 Minutes

Cook Time: 20 Minutes

Yield: serves 8

Ingredients

- 2 eggs
- 2 tablespoons sour cream
- generous pinch salt
- cracked pepper
- 2 teaspoons olive oil or butter
- 2 toasted 6 inch tortillas (corn or flour – or a mix)
- handful arugula or other greens
- one medium tomato diced- or slice cherry tomatoes in halves
- optional additions- sliced avocado, cilantro, browned meat/ chorizo /sausage, cheese, hot sauce, warmed seasoned black beans

Instructions

1. Heat oil in a non-stick pan or well-seasoned cast iron skillet over medium heat.

2. Whisk eggs with sour cream, salt and pepper.

3. Pour into a warm pan and gently stir- with a heat proof rubber or silicone spatula. As soon as soft lump of eggs begin to form, lower the heat to low and shift from stirring to folding the eggs over on themselves while gently shaking the pan with the other hand. Cook until desired done-ness. Turn heat off.

4. At the same time as cooking the eggs, place tortillas in a toaster oven until warmed through. You could also grill over a gas flame on the stove top using tongs.

5. Fold the warm fluffy eggs into warmed tortillas, top with arugula, tomatoes, a sprinkle of salt, and any optional additions, and a squirt of hot sauce. Eat immediately!

7. Mexican Breakfast Bowls

Prep Time: 150 Minutes

Cook Time: 20 Minutes

Yield: serves 8

Ingredients

- ½ an onion- diced
- 1 sweet potatoes (or yams) – diced into ½ inch cubes -about 2 cups
- 2 tablespoons oil
- generous pinch salt, pepper, chili powder
- 1 ½ cups cooked black beans (or one can drained), heated and seasoned with 1 teaspoon cumin, chili powder and a pinch of salt.
- 2 cups Turkey Chorizo (optional) or sub regular chorizo or vegan chorizo
- 4 Eggs
- Garnish: Avocado, cilantro, scallions, hot sauce, sour cream
- Other toppings: diced tomato, sautéed bell pepper or zucchini or other veggies

Instructions

1. Toss onion and sweet potato with the oil, season with salt, pepper and chili powder and roast on a parchment lined baking sheet in a 400F oven until tender, about 20 minutes. (Alternatively, sear in a skillet over medium heat, stirring occasionally for 10-15 minutes.)
2. If making chorizo, cook it with a little oil, browning it and breaking it apart into crumbles.
3. Heat the black beans, season with salt, chili pepper, and cumin.
4. Prepare the eggs to your liking– either scrambled, over easy, sunny side up, or poached.
5. Once the sweet potatoes are cooked, divide among 4 bowls. Divide the chorizo and black beans. Top with the eggs, avocado slices, cilantro and scallions. Add fresh tomatoes if in season.
6. Serve with your favorite hot sauce and a dollop of sour cream.

8. Succotash with Poached Eggs and Herb Oil

Prep Time: 15 Minutes

Cook Time: 30 Minutes

Yield: serves 4

Ingredients

- 1–2 tablespoons olive oil (or butter)
- 1 cup diced onion
- 3–4 rough chopped garlic cloves
- 2 cups diced Zucchini (or summer squash)
- 1 cup fresh green beans , sliced ½ inch pieces (or use okra, lima beans, or edamame)
- 1 red bell pepper, diced
- 2 ears of corn, shucked and kernels removed (about 2 cups)
- ¾ teaspoon smoked paprika
- ¾ teaspoon cumin
- ½ teaspoon salt
- ¼ teaspoon cracked pepper

- 4–8 large eggs, poached (or make crispy tofu!)

Herb Oil:

- ½ cup, packed finely chopped tender herbs (Italian parsley, tarragon, basil, cilantro, sage, oregano)
- 1 large garlic clove
- 1 tablespoon Lemon zest, chopped
- ½ cup olive oil
- 1/8 tsp salt, pepper, more to taste
- chile flakes (optional)
- Garnish
- fresh cherry tomatoes, sliced in half

Instructions

1. In a large skillet, heat oil over medium-high heat. Add onion. Saute until tender, about 3-4 minutes, add garlic.
2. Turn heat down to medium, and cook until garlic is fragrant about 2 minutes. Add zucchini and green beans and cook about 3-4 minutes, then turn heat to med low.
3. Add peppers and corn. Cooking on medium-low for 10-15 minutes until everything is tender. Season

with smoked paprika, salt, cumin and pepper. Taste adjusting salt and spices to your liking. You could add a splash of water to loosen.

4. Make the herb oil. Finely chop the herbs and garlic. Zest the lemon and chop it up a bit. Place all ingredients in a bowl and stir to combine. I prefer using mostly Italian parsley and then adding 1 or 2 other herbs as an accent. It takes quite a lot of herbs to make ½ cup chopped (it really condenses down, once chopped.)

5. Poach the eggs to the desired doneness.

6. Heat up the succotash (if necessary), loosen with a little water if you like- place the poached eggs over top and sprinkle with salt and pepper and a teaspoonful of the flavorful herb oil. Finish with aleppo chili flakes (or chili flakes).

7. Scatter with fresh cherry tomatoes over and around. Serve immediately.

9. Creamy Polenta with Eggs, Chorizo and Cilantro

Prep Time: 20 Minutes

Cook Time: 10 Minutes

Yield: serves 4

Ingredients

- 8 oz chorizo (links or ground) browned (or make this or use vegan chorizo)
- ¾ Cup dry polenta or corn meal
- 2 ½ C chicken stock (or veggie stock)
- 1 Cup grated melting cheese (mozzarella, cheddar, jack)
- ¼ C chopped cilantro divided
- ½ tsp smoked paprika
- salt and pepper to taste
- 6 eggs
- hot sauce for garnish
- variations- see below

Instructions

1. Pre-heat oven to 400F.

2. In a cast iron or oven proof 10 inch skillet, brown sausage or chorizo. Set aside.

3. In the same pan, add stock and bring to a boil. Turn heat to med low, whisk in polenta and smoked paprika, whisking vigorously -to prevent clumping. Once whisked well, cover, turn heat to low and let cook 15 minutes, stirring a few times.

4. Add grated cheese, stir to incorporate. Fold in ½ of the chopped cilantro, ½ of the browned chorizo (or sausage). Taste for salt and add if necessary.(If using chicken stock and chorizo, they will naturally be salty, but you may need to adjust- polenta should be flavorful.) Pepper to taste.

5. Place the other half of the chorizo on top of the polenta, in the center. With a spoon, make small wells in the polenta where the eggs will rest, around the outer edges of the skillet, in a circle. Crack the eggs and place them in the wells. Lightly salt and pepper each egg. Place the skillet in the 400F oven and bake until egg whites are white and set and yolks are set, but still soft (or cook until your desired doneness) .

6. I will often broil for just a quick minute. Garnish with hot sauce and remaining cilantro.

7. Note- You could add a bed sautéed spinach, sautéed peppers, sautéed onions, sautéed mushrooms to this dish, by placing atop the polenta and under the eggs. To get the calories down, leave out the chorizo.

10. Herby Smashed Potatoes

Prep Time: 15 Minutes

Cook Time: 45 Minutes

Yield: serves 4

Ingredients

- 1 1/2– 2 lbs thin-skinned potatoes (red, purple, golden, Yukons, fingerlings, etc.), steamed and cooled.
- 4 tablespoons olive oil (divided)
- 6 garlic cloves, smashed
- 1/4 cup herbs- rosemary, thyme, sage, or a combo
- Salt and pepper to taste
- Chili pepper or Aleppo Chili Flakes to taste

Instructions

1. Place whole potatoes in a large pot and cover with an inch of salted water. Bring to a boil, cover, lower heat and simmer until fork-tender, 20-30 minutes, depending on size. You want these fairly tender, so

they are easy to smash. Drain,let cool. You can do this the night before or few days before and store in the fridge. FYI Chilling potatoes after cooking actually increases health benefits (see post).

2. When ready to fry, heat oven to 400F (to keep the potatoes warm)

3. Smash the potatoes until relatively flattened, about 3/4 inch thick, using a potato masher or bottom of a skillet, set aside.

4. Heat 2-3 tablespoons olive oil in a cast-iron skillet over medium heat. Add the smashed garlic cloves and swirl the oil around, until fragrant and garlic is golden. Add the herbs, and cook for 45-60 seconds, infusing the oil. Set both aside, saving for the garnish at the end.

5. Season the fragrant rosemary garlic oil in the pan, with salt and pepper, and swirl.

6. Add the smashed potatoes, working in batches, leaving room to maneuver. Season the top of them with salt and pepper. Fry each side of the potatoes until crispy and deeply golden, about 5-7 minutes, resisting the urge to fiddle too much so they get nice and crispy. Add more oil if you need it when you flip.

7. Keep the first batch warm in the oven, while doing the second batch. When done, pile them up in the skillet.

8. Chop up the caramelized garlic cloves sprinkling along with the herbs over the potatoes.

9. Add chili flakes if you like and serve.

11. Tender, Golden Venezulean Corn Pancakes

Prep Time: 10 Minutes

Cook Time: 45 Minutes

Yield: serves 4

Ingredients

- 20 ounces frozen corn kernels (about 4 cups)
- 2 large eggs
- 1/2 cup whole milk
- 3 tablespoons vegetable oil
- 2 teaspoons salt
- 1 teaspoon granulated sugar
- 1/2 cup all-purpose flour
- 1 teaspoon baking powder
- 8 ounces fresh mozzarella cheese
- 6 teaspoons unsalted butter, divided

Instructions

1. Thaw 20 ounces frozen corn kernels overnight in the refrigerator or according to package directions. Drain well.

2. Transfer to a food processor fitted with a blade attachment. Add 2 large eggs, 1/2 cup whole milk, 3 tablespoons vegetable oil, 2 teaspoons kosher salt, and 1 teaspoon granulated sugar. Process until the mixture is a coarse purée, about 1 minute. Add 1/2 cup all-purpose flour and 1 teaspoon baking powder. Pulse until the flour is incorporated, about 1 minute. Transfer to a medium bowl.

3. Drain and thinly slice 8 ounces fresh mozzarella cheese (about 1/4-inch thick).

4. Melt 1 teaspoon of the unsalted butter in a 6-inch nonstick skillet over medium heat. Add 1/2 cup of the batter and smooth the top with the back of a spoon. Cover and cook until the bottom is golden-brown and the top is no longer wet, 4 to 6 minutes.

5. Uncover and add a few slices of the mozzarella to one half of the cachapa. Fold the other half over the cheese. Cover and cook until the cheese is melted, about 1 minute. Transfer the cachapa to a plate or platter. Repeat cooking the remaining batter, melting

1 teaspoon unsalted butter in the pan before each cachapa. If the butter starts to brown, reduce the heat slightly and wipe the skillet clean between each cachapa. Because these cachapas are extremely tender and custardy, they are best eaten right away.

12. Caprese Sandwich

Prep Time: 30 Minutes

Cook Time: 25 Minutes

Yield: serves 6

Ingredients

- 20–24 inch baguette
- 3–4 tablespoons pesto- store-bought, arugula pesto or Basil Pesto
- 1/4 cup mayo
- 3–4 ripe tomatoes, medium
- 1–2 large mozzarella balls, sliced
- 10 basil leaves
- salt and pepper
- drizzle of olive oil
- drizzle of balsamic vinegar, or balsamic glaze
- Arugula Pesto (makes one cup)
- 2 large garlic cloves
- 1/4 cup smoked almonds (or toasted almonds, or pinenuts)
- 1 cup packed Basil leaves (or flat-leaf parsley)

- 2 cups packed Arugula
- 1/2 cup olive oil
- 1/8 cup fresh lemon juice
- 1/4–1/2 tsp kosher salt (if your almonds are heavily salted, use salt to taste.)
- cracked pepper

Instructions

1. Make arugula pesto if using: Place everything in a food processor and pulse repeatedly, until uniformly combined, but not too smooth.
2. Slice baguette in half lengthwise, leaving one side intact. Toast it a little if you like.
3. Mix the 1/4 cup mayo and 3-4 tablespoons pesto together. Slather over the insides of the baguette.
4. Layer with mozzarella and tomatoes. Season with salt and pepper.
5. Add the fresh basil. Drizzle with olive oil and balsamic.
6. Close the baguette and cut it into 5- 6 pieces. Tightly wrap any leftovers and keep in the fridge for up to 2-3 days.

13. Homemade Bread Is Made with Ground Sausage Rolled in Pizza Dough

Prep Time: 40 Minutes

Cook Time: 45 Minutes

Yield: serves 8

Ingredients

- 1 pound pizza dough
- 1 small shallot
- 4 ounces baby bella or cremini mushrooms
- 2 cloves garlic
- 3 tablespoons olive oil, divided
- 2 teaspoons Italian seasoning
- 1 to 2 teaspoons red pepper flakes
- 1 teaspoon salt
- 1 teaspoon freshly ground black pepper
- 1 pound uncooked sweet or spicy Italian sausage, casings removed if needed
- All-purpose flour, for stretching out the dough
- 2 cups shredded Italian cheese blend (4 ounces)

- 1 large egg
- 1 tablespoon grated Parmesan cheese (optional)
- Marinara sauce, for serving

Instructions

1. If pizza dough is refrigerated, let it sit on the counter until it comes to room temperature, about 2 hours.
2. Arrange a rack in the middle of the oven and heat the oven to 425°F.
3. Finely chop 1 small shallot (1/4 cup), 4 ounces baby bella mushrooms, and 2 garlic cloves. Beat 1 large egg in a small bowl.
4. Heat 2 tablespoons of the olive oil in a large skillet over medium-high heat until shimmering. Add the shallots, mushrooms, and garlic and cook, stirring occasionally, until the shallots are translucent and the mushrooms are lightly browned, 5 to 8 minutes.
5. Reduce the heat to medium-low. Add 2 teaspoons Italian seasoning, 1 to 2 teaspoons red pepper flakes (depending on spice preference), 1 teaspoon kosher salt, and 1 teaspoon black pepper. Cook until fragrant, about 2 minutes more. Transfer to a large bowl.

6. Return the skillet to medium-high heat and heat the remaining 1 tablespoon olive oil in the pan until shimmering. Add 1 pound Italian sausage and cook, breaking up the meat into small pieces and stirring occasionally, until browned and cooked through, 7 to 8 minutes. Drain on a paper towel-lined plate, then add to the mushroom mixture and stir to combine.

7. Dust a large sheet of parchment paper with all-purpose flour, then place the pizza dough on top. Stretch and roll the dough out to a 12x9-inch rectangle about 1/4-inch thick. Don't roll the dough out too thin or the filling will spill out once rolled. It's OK if the dough doesn't form a perfect rectangle — having an even thickness is more important.

8. Spread the meat mixture on top, leaving a 1/2-inch border, then sprinkle with 2 cups shredded Italian cheese blend. Starting from a shorter end, roll the dough up tightly. Tuck the ends underneath and position seam-side down.

9. Transfer the parchment paper with the rolled-up dough onto a baking sheet. Cut 4 (2-inch) slits into the top of the dough. Brush the dough with the egg, then sprinkle with 1 tablespoon grated Parmesan cheese if desired.

10. Bake until the bread is golden-brown and cooked through, 30 to 35 minutes. Let cool for 10 minutes before slicing. Serve with marinara sauce for dipping.

14. Lentil Bolognese

Prep Time: 20 Minutes

Cook Time: 45 Minutes

Yield: serves 8

Ingredients

- 2 tablespoons olive oil
- 1 large onion, diced
- 1 1/2 cup carrots, small diced
- 1 1/2 cups celery diced
- 4–6 cloves garlic, rough chopped
- 1 1/2 teaspoon salt
- 1/2 teaspoon pepper
- 1/4 teaspoon chili flakes- optional
- 1 tablespoon fresh oregano or thyme (or 2 teaspoons dried Italian herbs)
- 1/3 cup tomato paste
- Generous splash red wine (optional) 1/4 cup-ish
- 1 1/4 cup black caviar lentils (or other small lentils- see notes)

- 3 medium tomatoes, diced with juices (or sub a 14-ounce can of diced tomatoes or crushed tomatoes)
- 3 1/2 cups veggie stock or broth (or sub water plus 2-3 boullion cubes)
- 3/4 cup hemp seeds, or crushed toasted walnuts or pecans
- 2 teaspoons balsamic vinegar

Instructions

1. Heat oil in a large pot or dutch oven over medium-high heat. Add the onion and saute for 2-3 minutes stirring until fragrant. Lower heat to medium, then add the carrots, celery, garlic, salt, pepper, chili flakes, and herbs. Saute 7-8 minutes, stirring.

2. Add the tomato paste, browning it just a bit in the pan (this will deepen the flavor), then deglaze with wine if you want, scraping up any brown bits. Once most of the wine has cooked off add the tomatoes and their juices, cook them down for just a few minutes.

3. Add the lentils, veggie stock and hemp seeds or walnuts. Bring to a boil, cover tightly,

lower heat to low, and simmer gently 20-25 minutes, or until the lentils are tender. Uncover.

4. Continue cooking uncovered until most of the liquid has cooked off. Stir in the balsamic vinegar, taste, and adjust salt, pepper, vinegar and chili flakes to your liking. Keep in mind, you want this just slightly salty if tossing with pasta.

5. Serve this tossed with your favorite pasta or serve it over this creamy polenta or this Instant Pot Polenta. Sprinkle with optional pecorino cheese... or try this Vegan Cheesy Sprinkle!

15. Classic Deli Turkey Salad Tossed in A Mayo-Based

Prep Time: 20 Minutes

Cook Time: 45 Minutes

Yield: serves 8

Ingredients

- 1 tablespoon avocado or canola oil
- 1/4 cup shelled pumpkin seeds
- 1/4 cup slivered almonds
- 2 tablespoons white sesame seeds
- 1/2 bunch fresh cilantro
- 3 medium scallions
- 1 large (or 2 small) canned chipotles in adobo sauce
- 1/2 medium lime
- 1/4 cup mayonnaise
- 1/4 cup sour cream
- 1/2 teaspoon salt
- 1/4 teaspoon freshly ground black pepper
- 16 ounces cooked and shredded turkey (about 4 cups)

Instructions

1. Heat 1 tablespoon avocado oil in a small frying pan over medium-low heat. Add 1/4 cup pumpkin seeds and 1/4 cup slivered almonds to the pan. Cook and stir until the pumpkin seeds start to pop, 1 to 3 minutes. Add 2 tablespoons white sesame seeds. Cook, stirring often, until the sesame seeds start to brown, 1 to 2 minutes. Remove the pan from the heat and set aside to cool while you prepare the remaining ingredients.

2. Finely chop 1/2 bunch fresh cilantro until you have 1/4 cup. Thinly slice 3 medium scallions (1/4 cup).

3. Finely chop 1 large or 2 small chipotles in adobo sauce until you have 2 tablespoons and place in a large bowl. Squeeze the juice from 1/2 medium lime (1 tablespoon) into the bowl. Add 1/4 cup mayonnaise, 1/4 cup sour cream, 1/2 teaspoon kosher salt, and 1/4 teaspoon black pepper, and whisk to combine.

4. Add the cilantro, scallions, cooled nuts and seeds, and 2 cups cooked and shredded turkey. Use a spatula or large spoon to coat the turkey in the dressing.

16. Moroccan Lentil and Chickpea Soup

Prep Time: 20 Minutes

Cook Time: 45 Minutes

Yield: serves 10

Ingredients

- 2 tablespoons olive oil
- 1 onion, diced
- 2 stalks of celery, inner leaves are fine, chopped small
- 4 cloves garlic, chopped
- 1 1/2 teaspoons dried ground ginger
- 1/2 teaspoon black pepper
- 1/2 teaspoon turmeric
- 2 teaspoons cumin
- 1 teaspoon smoked paprika
- 1/4–1/2 teaspoon cayenne
- 6 cups broth, vegetable or chicken or water
- 1 28 ounce canned, whole or crushed tomatoes
- 1 cinnamon stick (or 1/4 teaspoon ground cinnamon)

- a tiny pinch of saffron (optional)
- 1–2 teaspoons sea salt
- 1/2 cup red lentils
- 1/2 cup brown or green lentils
- 1 1/2 cups or 1 15- ounce can of chickpeas (garbanzo beans)
- 2 teaspoons honey (if needed)
- 1/4 pound capellini pasta, broken into approximately 1-inch pieces
- 1/2 cup chopped cilantro, stems are great
- 1/2 cup parsley
- Serve with lemon wedges, a swirl of yogurt (if desired) and dates on the side.

Instructions

1. Saute onions for 5 minutes in olive oil, over medium heat.
2. Add celery, garlic, ginger, pepper, turmeric, cumin, smoked paprika and cayenne. Stir for another minute. Sautéing the spices allows them to bloom and deepen in flavor.
3. Add broth, tomatoes, cinnamon sticks, saffron, salt, red lentils, brown lentils, half of

the cilantro and half of the parsley. Bring to a
simmer, cover with a vented lid, for 30 minutes.

4. Add Chickpeas and pasta cook 5-10 minutes more.
    (see notes)

5. Add honey and remaining fresh herbs.

17. Dijon Mustard and Tangy Sauerkraut

Prep Time: 20 Minutes

Cook Time: 45 Minutes

Yield: serves 10

Ingredients

- 1 large egg
- 1 cup drained sauerkraut (about 4 1/2 ounces)
- 1 (8-ounce) can refrigerated crescent roll dough
- 4 tablespoons whole-grain mustard, divided
- 4 fully cooked bratwurst sausages (about 12 ounces total)
- 2 teaspoons everything bagel spice (optional), divided

Instructions

1. Arrange a rack in the middle of the oven and heat the oven to 400°F. Line a baking sheet with parchment paper or silicone baking mat. Place 1 large egg in a small bowl and whisk with a fork until no streaks of egg white remain.

2. Spread 1 cup drained sauerkraut out on a double layer of paper towels. Roll up into a log and squeeze as much liquid out as you can. Transfer the sauerkraut to a cutting board and coarsely chop.

3. Unroll 1 can crescent roll dough on a work surface and separate into 4 rectangles (2 triangles each). Press on the seams in each rectangle to seal. Spread 1 tablespoon whole-grain mustard on each rectangle, then sprinkle with the sauerkraut.

4. Place 1 bratwurst sausage on a short end of each rectangle. Starting at the end with the bratwurst, roll up tightly. Place seam-side down on the baking sheet. Brush the top and the sides of each one with the egg wash. Cut 3 parallel 1-inch slits into the top dough of each pig in a blanket. Sprinkle each one with 1/2 teaspoon everything bagel spice if desired.

5. Bake until deep golden-brown, 15 to 18 minutes. Let cool for 5 minutes before serving.

18. Navy Bean Soup

Prep Time: 20 Minutes

Cook Time: 50 Minutes

Yield: serves 6

Ingredients

- 1 pound dried navy beans
- 4 cups hot water
- 1 medium yellow onion
- 1 large carrot
- 1 stalk celery
- 2 cloves garlic
- 8 ounces thick-cut cooked ham
- 2 tablespoons olive oil
- 2 bay leaves
- 2 teaspoons freshly ground black pepper
- 1 teaspoon salt, plus more as needed
- 1/2 teaspoon dried thyme
- 1/2 teaspoon dried rosemary
- 1 smoked ham hock (optional)
- 6 cups low-sodium chicken broth

- 2 tablespoons unsalted butter

Instructions

1. Rinse 1 pound dried navy beans and remove and discard split, broken, or discolored beans. Place the beans and 4 cups hot water in a large, heavy pot or Dutch oven. Bring to a boil over medium-high heat. Boil for 2 minutes, then remove the pot from heat. Cover and let soak for 1 hour.

2. Meanwhile, finely chop 1 medium yellow onion (1 1/2 to 2 cups), 1 large carrot (1/2 cup), and 1 medium celery stalk (1/2 cup). Finely chop 2 garlic cloves. Dice 8 ounces thick-cut cooked ham (1 cup).

3. When the beans are done soaking, pour through a colander to drain. Wipe the pot clean.

4. Heat 2 tablespoons olive oil in the same pot over medium heat until shimmering. Add the onion, carrot, and celery, and cook, stirring occasionally, until fragrant and begin to soften, about 3 minutes. Add the ham, garlic, 2 bay leaves, 2 teaspoons black pepper, 1 teaspoon kosher salt, 1/2 teaspoon dried thyme, and 1/2 teaspoon dried rosemary. Sauté until fragrant, about 1 minute.

5. Add the beans and stir to combine. If desired, nestle 1 smoked ham hock into the bean mixture. Add 6 cups low-sodium chicken broth and bring to a boil over high heat. Reduce the heat to medium-low and simmer gently, stirring occasionally, until the beans are tender, 1 hour 30 minutes to 1 hour 45 minutes.

6. Remove the ham hock. Add 2 tablespoons unsalted butter and stir until melted. Taste and season with more kosher salt as needed.

19. Soba Noodle Salad

Prep Time: 20 Minutes

Cook Time: 15 Minutes

Yield: serves 6

Ingredients

Dressing:

- 2 tablespoons toasted sesame oil
- 1/4 cup tamari, soy sauce or Bragg's liquid amino acids
- 1/4 cup rice wine vinegar
- 1 tablespoons mirin
- 2 teaspoons sugar

Salad:

- 8 ounces buckwheat soba noodles
- 1 ½ cups English cucumber, sliced in half moons or diced
- 2 cups Bok Choy (or napa cabbage or green cabbage), shredded
- 1 colored bell pepper, cut in small strips

- 1 cup snow peas, chopped
- ½ cups sliced green onion, chopped fine
- 1 cup mixed herbs, dill cilantro mint, roughly chopped
- 2 tablespoons toasted sesame seeds
- 4 oz Smoked Salmon or baked tofu (optional)

Instructions

1. Whisk together the dressing. Combine the sesame oil, soy sauce, rice vinegar, mirin and sugar.
2. Cook soba noodles, according to package directions, (about 4-6 minutes) in plenty of boiling salted water. Drain, rinse with lots of cold water, place in medium bowl.
3. Add prepped veggies into the noodles and toss with the dressing.
4. Sprinkle toasted sesame seeds on top.
5. If desired top with smoked tofu or smoked salmon.
6. Optional Garnishes: dulse seaweed flakes, chili flakes, black sesame seeds and sriracha.

20. Creamy Broccoli Soup with Pesto

Prep Time: 20 Minutes

Cook Time: 15 Minutes

Yield: serves 6

Ingredients

- 1 1/2 lbs broccoli, stems too!
- 2 tablespoons olive oil (or butter, or ghee)
- 1 white or yellow onion, diced
- 4–6 garlic cloves, rough chopped
- 3 cups veggie broth or chicken stock, divided (or use water and 2–3 teaspoons- Better than Boullion)
- 1 cup almond milk (or cashew milk, whole milk or half and half)
- 1/2 cup fresh basil
- 1/2-1 teaspoon salt
- Pepper to taste
- Pinch cayenne (optional)
- 1/4 cup plain yogurt or sour cream (feel free to use vegan, or a splash of heavy cream), more to taste.

- Garnish: Pesto (store-bought, Homemade Pesto, or Arugula pesto), Parmesan Crisps, Vegan Cheesy Sprinkle

Instructions

1. Thinly slice the broccoli stems and break apart the florets into very small pieces. Chop the onion and garlic.
2. In a heavy bottom pot or dutch oven, heat the oil over medium heat. Saute the onion and garlic with a pinch of salt, until golden and fragrant, about 4-5 minutes.
3. Add the broccoli stems, and pour in the stock or broth and bring to boil. Cover, lower heat, and simmer gently 3-4 minutes.
4. Place the broccoli florets over the top. Don't mix them in. Cover, and simmer gently, allowing the florets to steam, until fork-tender, about 5 minutes. You want them tender enough to blend but not overly cooked or you'll lose that vibrant color.
5. Turn the heat off. Blend in two batches (I found using a blender was better here, my immersion blender did not work as well) adding half of the

almond milk to each batch, along with the basil. Blend until smooth. Add a handful of spinach for richer color if you like.

6. Return the soup to the pot and stir in the yogurt or sour cream or even a splash of heavy cream. Gently warm the soup and season with salt and pepper to taste.

7. Serve with a swirl of pesto, crusty bread, or Parmesan crips. Enjoy!

21. Pan-Roasted Chicken with Grapes

Prep Time: 20 Minutes

Cook Time: 30 Minutes

Yield: serves 4

Ingredients

- 1 tablespoon olive oil
- 1 garlic clove, smashed
- 4 chicken thighs, skin-on, bone-in
- salt and pepper to taste
- 3 fat shallots, sliced lengthwise
- 1 tablespoon balsamic vinegar (sherry vinegar, or apple cider vinegar, or any flavorful complementary vinegar)
- 1 lb seedless grapes (red), divided into small clusters
- 1 tablespoon chopped rosemary
- Serve with Ginger Whipped Sweet Potatoes

Instructions

1. Preheat oven to 400F

2. If making the Ginger Whipped Sweet Potatoes, get them simmering in a pot.

3. Heat oil in an oven-proof skillet over medium high heat. Add smashed garlic clove and swirl, to season the oil. Season the skin side of the chicken generously, with salt and pepper, and place skin side down in hot skillet. Season the other side of chicken with salt and pepper, and remove the garlic. Sear skin side until golden and crispy, 6-7 minutes, turning heat to medium. Flip. Place the shallots between the chicken and drizzle with the vinegar. Top with the grape clusters, nestling between and around the chicken. Sprinkle with rosemary and place in the oven for 20 minutes or until internal temp reaches 170F.

4. While it's baking, finish making the ginger whipped sweet potatoes.

5. When chicken seems done, place skillet back the stove and bring it to a quick simmer (just to make sure juices are cooked.) Spoon the whipped sweet potatoes onto plates, top with crispy chicken and

divide shallots and grapes among the plates. Spoon some flavorful pan sauce over everything.

6. Enjoy!

22. Cheesy-Filled Pasta Even Cheesier

Prep Time: 20 Minutes

Cook Time: 30 Minutes

Yield: serves 4

Ingredients

- 4 ounces Parmesan cheese (2 cups loosely packed grated or 1 cup store-bought grated)
- 3 cloves garlic
- 4 tablespoons (1/2 stick) unsalted butter
- 1 1/2 cups half-and-half
- 3/4 teaspoon salt, plus more as needed Freshly ground black pepper
- 18 to 20 ounces fresh or frozen cheese tortellini (do not thaw)
- Finely chopped fresh parsley leaves, for garnish (optional)

Instructions

1. Bring a large pot of heavily salted water to a boil over medium-high heat. Meanwhile, make the sauce.

2. Finely grate 4 ounces Parmesan cheese on the smallest holes of a box grater if needed (about 2 loosely packed cups), or measure out 1 cup store-bought grated. Finely grate or mince 3 garlic cloves (about 1 tablespoon). Melt 4 tablespoons unsalted butter in a large frying pan or skillet (preferably nonstick) over medium heat. Add the garlic and cook until fragrant but not browned, about 30 seconds.

3. Add 1 1/2 cups half-and-half and bring to a simmer. Add the cheese, 3/4 teaspoon kosher salt, and a few grinds of black pepper. Whisk to combine and bring to a simmer. Turn off the heat.

4. Add the tortellini to the boiling water and cook, stirring occasionally, for 2 minutes less than package directions. Reserve 1/2 cup of the pasta water. Drain the pasta.

5. Add the pasta to the sauce and cook over medium heat, stirring often, until heated through and the sauce thickens slightly, about 2 minutes. Add some of the pasta water to thin out the sauce if needed. Taste and season with more kosher salt and black pepper as

needed. Garnish with finely chopped fresh parsley leaves if desired.

23. Classic with Loads Of Bacon

Prep Time: 20 Minutes

Cook Time: 30 Minutes

Yield: serves 4

Ingredients

- 10 to 12 slices bacon (10 to 12 ounces), divided
- 3/4 cup ketchup
- 2 tablespoons packed dark or light brown sugar
- 1 teaspoon smoked paprika
- 1 small yellow onion
- 2 pounds lean ground beef (90% lean)
- 1/2 cup plain fine breadcrumbs
- 2 large eggs
- 1 tablespoon Worcestershire sauce
- 1 teaspoon kosher salt
- 1/2 teaspoon freshly ground black pepper
- 1/2 teaspoon garlic powder

Instructions

1. Arrange a rack in the middle of the oven and heat the
    oven to 350°F.

2. Line the bottom and sides of a 9x5-inch loaf pan with
    8 to 10 slices of the bacon, overlapping them slightly
    to cover and letting them hang over the top slightly.

3. Place 3/4 cup ketchup, 2 tablespoons packed brown
    sugar, and 1 teaspoon smoked paprika in a small bowl
    and stir to combine. Transfer 1/4 cup into the pan and
    spread evenly over the bottom.

4. Finely chop 1 small yellow onion until you have 1 cup
    and place in a large bowl. Add 2 pounds lean ground
    beef, 1/2 cup plain breadcrumbs, 2 large eggs, 1
    tablespoon Worcestershire sauce, 1 teaspoon kosher
    salt, 1/2 teaspoon black pepper, and 1/2 teaspoon
    garlic powder. Mix with your hands until well
    combined, but do not overmix.

5. Transfer to the pan and pat into an even layer. Fold
    the overhanging bacon over the top of the meatloaf.

6. Line a rimmed baking sheet with aluminum foil.
    Invert the baking sheet over the loaf pan. Holding
    both the baking sheet and the loaf pan, flip both over
    in one motion. Remove the loaf pan to unmold the
    meatloaf.

7. Cut the remaining 2 bacon slices in half crosswise. Press 2 pieces onto each end of the meatloaf to cover the ends. Tuck the pieces under the other bacon to hold them in place.

8. Bake for 50 minutes. Remove the meatloaf from the oven. Brush the top, sides, and ends with the remaining ketchup mixture. Return to the oven and bake until cooked through and an instant-read thermometer inserted into the center registers at least 165°F, about 30 minutes more. Let the meatloaf rest for 10 minutes before slicing and serving.

24.Baked Chicken Shawarma (Vegan Adaptable!)

Prep Time: 15 Minutes

Cook Time: 30 Minutes

Yield: serves 4 Cups

Ingredients

- 1– 1 ½ pounds chicken (breast or thigh) or tofu or a mix of both (like 1 pound chicken and 8 ounces tofu)
- 1 onion
- 1 red pepper- optional
- 1 cauliflower – optional see notes
- Quick Shawarma Marinade:
- 1 teaspoon kosher salt
- 2 teaspoons cumin
- 2 teaspoons coriander
- 1 teaspoon turmeric
- 1 teaspoon granulated garlic (or two cloves, finely minced)

- 2 tablespoons olive oil

Wrap Options:

- 4 x 10-12 inch wraps or pita bread
- Cucumber, radish, or tomato, Everyday Kale Slaw or Isreali Salad or greens like arugula or spinach
- Shawarma Bowl Options:
- cooked grain (rice, quinoa, barley) or roasted, "riced" cauliflower (see notes)
- roasted cauliflower or other roasted veggies
- Serve both with Everyday Tahini Sauce, Zhoug, or Zhoug Yogurt, Baba ganoush and optional Isreali Salad.

Instructions

1. Preheat oven to 400 F
2. Whisk the marinade ingredients together in a small bowl.
3. On a large parchment lined sheet-pan, place chicken breasts, tofu filets, and any vegetables that you want to use. Brush the chicken and tofu very liberally with marinade. For the other veggies,

drizzle with olive oil, salt, pepper and a little lemon zest is nice. ☐ Place in the oven for 20-30 minutes.

4. If making a grain bowl, cook the grains now. You could also roast "riced" cauliflower at the same time, on another sheet pan. Season it with olive oil, salt, pepper, lemon zest, perhaps some cumin – toss it every 10 minutes or so until cooked with a few nice crispy bits.

5. Check chicken after 20 minutes (breast will cook faster). Toss veggies, and cook until chicken is cooked through and veggies are tender. Tofu takes 30 minutes to get a nice crust.

6. Cut chicken and assemble bowls or make the wraps. Drizzle with Tahini sauce and/or Zhoug yogurt.

7. If making wraps, use a warm tortillas or warm pita. Add greens, pickled onions, crunchy veggies, greens or kale   slaw,   and   spoon tahini   sauce over top. Zhoug yogurt is nice too!

25. Croque Monsieur

Prep Time: 15 Minutes

Cook Time: 30 Minutes

Yield: serves 4 Cups

Ingredients

For the béchamel:

- 2 tablespoons unsalted butter
- 2 tablespoons all-purpose flour
- 3/4 cup whole or 2% milk
- 2 teaspoons regular or whole-grain Dijon mustard
- 1/8 teaspoon ground nutmeg
- 1/8 teaspoon salt
- 1/8 teaspoon freshly ground black pepper

For assembly:

- 8 (1/2-inch thick) slices pan de mie, country-style sourdough bread, or hearty white sandwich bread
- 6 to 8 ounces sliced unsmoked ham (about 8 slices)
- 6 ounces Gruyère cheese

Instructions

1. Arrange a rack in the upper third of the oven and heat the oven to 425°F.
2. Make the bechamel:
3. Melt 2 tablespoons unsalted butter in a small saucepan over medium heat. Add 2 tablespoons all-purpose flour and whisk until combined, about 1 minute. While whisking constantly, slowly pour in 3/4 cup whole or 2% milk. Bring to a simmer (it will start to thicken up), whisking constantly.
4. Remove the saucepan from the heat. Add 2 teaspoons Dijon mustard, 1/8 teaspoon ground nutmeg, 1/8 teaspoon kosher salt, and 1/8 teaspoon black pepper, and whisk to combine.
5. Assemble the sandwiches:
6. Line a baking sheet with parchment paper. Grate 6 ounces Gruyère cheese on the large holes of a box grater(about 2 cups). Place 4 (1/2-inch) thick slices bread on the baking sheet. Spread 2 tablespoons béchamel on each slice of bread. Divide 6 to 8 ounces sliced ham over the béchamel, bending and folding then as needed to fit. Sprinkle half the cheese on top of the ham.

7. Close the sandwiches with the remaining 4 bread slices. Spread 2 tablespoons béchamel evenly onto each slice of bread. Sprinkle with the remaining cheese.

8. Bake until the edges of the bread are crispy and the tops are starting to brown, about 15 minutes. Heat the oven to broil. Broil until deep golden brown in spots, about 3 minutes more. Let cool for 5 minutes before serving.

26. Savory Mushroom Crepes with Spaghetti Squash and Sage

Prep Time: 5 Minutes

Cook Time: 60 Minutes

Yield: serves 4

Ingredients

Spaghetti Squash Filling :

- 1 smallish spaghetti squash (about 3 pounds)
- 1 tablespoon olive oil
- salt to taste
- black pepper to taste
- 1/2 onion, diced and sauteed (optional, or sub 1 shallot)
- ½ teaspoon fresh grated nutmeg (or pre-ground)
- 1 tablespoon chopped fresh sage leaves
- 1 teaspoon maple syrup
- 1/2 cup grated Parmigiano-Reggiano or Romano cheese

Crepes:

- 2 large eggs
- ½ cup milk
- ½ cup water
- 1 cup flour
- 2 tablespoons melted butter
- ¼ tsp kosher salt
- Butter, for coating the pan

Mushroom Topping:

- 1 T butter + 1 T olive oil
- 1 shallot, finely sliced
- 8 oz mushrooms- quartered or sliced (cremini, chanterelles, shiitake, morels, porcini)
- salt and pepper to taste
- 1–2 teaspoons chopped sage
- a drizzle of truffle oil– optional

Bechamel Sauce:

- 3 tablespoons butter
- 1/4 cup minced shallots (optional)
- 1/4 cup all-purpose flour
- 2 cups milk
- 1/8 teaspoon ground nutmeg
- 1/2 teaspoon kosher salt

Instructions

1. Start the filling: Heat the oven to 425°F and arrange a rack in the middle. Cut the squash in half lengthwise and scrape out the seeds. Brush the flesh with oil and season generously with salt and pepper. Place the squash halves cut-side down on a baking sheet and roast until fork-tender, about 35-45 minutes. (You could do this ahead.)

2. Make the crepes: In a large mixing bowl, whisk together the flour and the eggs. Gradually add in the milk and water, stirring to combine. Add the salt and melted butter; beat until smooth. Heat a lightly oiled or buttered 8-10 -inch frying pan over medium-high heat. Pour or scoop the batter onto the pan using approximately 1/4 cup for each crepe. Tilt the pan with a circular motion so that the batter coats the surface evenly. Cook the crepe for about 2 minutes, until the bottom is light brown. Loosen with a spatula, turn and cook the other side. Set aside and stack. (you could make these ahead and refrigerate, covering)

3. Make the Mushroom Topping: Saute the shallot and mushrooms in 1-2 T butter /oil until over medium heat until golden and tender and season

with salt and pepper and fresh sage. Drizzle with a teaspoon of truffle oil, if you like. Set aside.

4. Make the Bechamel Sauce. Melt butter in a small, heavy saucepan over medium heat until foaming. Add shallots (if using) and sauté 2 minutes. Do not let brown. Reduce heat to low, add flour, and whisk until smooth and raw taste is cooked off, about 1 minute. Gradually whisk in milk, starting with ½ cup, whisking well, then adding another half cup at a time until all is incorporated. Cook until just thickened, stirring often, about 10 minutes. Stir in nutmeg and salt. Season with ground white pepper. (You could make this ahead, refrigerate, and heat up (whisking) before serving. Loosen, if needed with a little milk or water.)

5. Make the Filling: Remove the squash from the oven and let sit at room temperature until cool enough to handle, about 10 minutes. Scrape the flesh with a fork to make long strands; place in a bowl. You should have about 4 cups. If there is more, save the extra for another use. Add nutmeg, maple syrup, white pepper, sage, sautéed onions (optional) and cheese and mix thoroughly, and

taste for salt, adding more to taste. (You could make this ahead.)

6. Assemble: Divide the squash filling among the crepes, and fold them over. (You could fill these ahead and refrigerate.) Heat ½ T butter and ½ T olive oil in a pan or skillet and fry each stuffed crepe on both sides until golden and crispy, adding more butter if necessary, and placing in a warm oven until all are crisped.

7. To plate, place two crispy crepes on top of each other and cut down the middle, so you have 4 triangles. Stack vertically on a plate and drizzle with béchamel sauce, top with sautéed mushrooms. Serve immediately.

27. Classic Italian Dish

Prep Time: 35 Minutes

Cook Time: 50 Minutes

Yield: serves 6

Ingredients

- 1 large lemon
- 2 large artichokes (10 to 12 ounces each)
- 2 large cloves garlic
- 2 cups panko breadcrumbs
- 3 ounces Parmesan cheese (about 1 1/2 firmly packed cups grated on a Microplane or 1 cup store-bought grated)
- 2 teaspoons Italian seasoning
- 1 teaspoon salt
- 1/2 teaspoon red pepper flakes
- 3/4 cup olive oil
- 2 teaspoons anchovy paste
- 1 bay leaf

Instructions

1. Finely grate the zest of 1 large lemon into a large bowl. Fill a large pot with enough water to submerge 2 large artichokes. (If you have a steamer pot, use the base of that one.) Cut the lemon in half, squeeze the juice into the water, and drop the juiced lemon halves into the water.

2. Slice the stems off of 2 large artichokes, peel them, and add to the lemon water. Slice off and discard 1 inch off the artichoke tops with a serrated knife. Use kitchen shears to snip off the thorny tips from the petals. Gently fan open the petals of each artichoke, working from the outside in until you reach the fuzzy chokes in the center. Scrape out the choke with a spoon and place the artichokes upside down in the lemon water to prevent them from darkening.

3. Mince 2 large garlic cloves and finely grate 3 ounces Parmesan cheese (about 1 1/2 packed cups) if needed. Add both to the lemon zest bowl. Add 2 cups panko breadcrumbs, 2 teaspoons Italian seasoning, 1 teaspoon kosher salt, and 1/2 teaspoon red pepper flakes. Stir until combined.

4. Pour 3/4 cup olive oil into a glass measuring cup and whisk in 2 teaspoons anchovy paste. Add the dressing to the breadcrumb mixture and mix well to combine.

5. Remove the artichokes from the water and shake off any excess water. Place right-side up on a work surface. Working with 1 artichoke at a time, stuff the breading into the center well and between every petal.

6. Add 1 bay leaf to the pot of lemon water and bring it to boil over meidum-high heat. Place the stuffed artichokes and stems in a steamer tray or basket and place in the pot, making sure the water does not touch the bottom of the tray. Cover and steam over medium-low heat, adding more water as needed, until tender, about 1 hour and 20 minutes. To test, tug on a petal and if it doesn't pull away easily, steam for 10 more minutes and try again.

7. Use tongs to transfer the artichokes to a platter. If you want some browning, place the stuffed artichokes on a baking sheet and broil in the oven until golden-brown, 2 to 3 minutes.

28. Zucchini, Corn and Basil Stir-Fry with Tofu, Shrimp or Chicken

Prep Time: 35 Minutes

Cook Time: 450 Minutes

Yield: serves 6

Ingredients

- 8 ounces tofu, shrimp, chicken breast or chicken sausage
- 1–2 tablespoon olive oil
- generous pinch salt and pepper
- ½ cup red onion, or 2 shallots
- 4 cups zucchini or summer squash, sliced into half moons or quarter moons, a ½ inch thick. (about 3 medium sized squash)
- 2 cloves garlic- rough chopped
- 1 ear of corn, kernels sliced off (or sub a fresh red bell pepper, diced)
- salt and pepper to taste
- ¼ cup fresh torn basil or basil ribbons

- aleppo chili flakes (optional)

Instructions

1. Heat oil in an extra large skillet or wok over medium high heat. Season the oil with generous pinch of salt and pepper and sear the tofu (cubed), shrimp or chicken (diced), turning heat down to medium if necessary, and cook until all sides are seared and cooked to your liking. Set aside.
2. To the same skillet, add a bit more oil if necessary and heat over medium-high heat. Add onion. Saute for 2 minutes until fragrant. Add zucchini. Continue cooking, stirring frequently for about 5 minutes until zucchini begins to turn golden.

29. Cottage Pie

Prep Time: 35 Minutes

Cook Time: 450 Minutes

Yield: serves 6

Ingredients

For the beef filling:

- 2 medium carrots
- 2 large stalks celery
- 1 large yellow onion
- 2 cloves garlic
- 3 tablespoons olive oil, divided
- 1 to 1 1/3 pounds lean ground beef
- 4 cups low-sodium beef broth, or 4 cups reconstituted beef bouillon paste or cubes and water (follow package directions)
- 1 1/2 teaspoons salt, divided
- 3 large sprigs fresh thyme
- 2 tablespoons tomato paste
- 1/4 cup all-purpose flour

- 1 cup dry red wine

- 1/4 cup Worcestershire sauce

- 1/2 teaspoon ground white pepper or freshly ground black pepper

- For the mashed potatoes:

- 2 1/2 pounds russet potatoes (4 to 5 medium)

- 2 bay leaves

- 2 1/2 teaspoons salt, divided

- 1/2 cup heavy cream, divided (optional)

- 3/4 cup whole milk

- 4 tablespoons (1/2 stick) unsalted butter

- 1/2 teaspoon ground white pepper or freshly ground black pepper

- 1 ounce aged cheddar or Parmesan cheese

Instructions

1. Peel 2 medium carrots and finely dice. Finely dice 2 large celery stalks and 1 large yellow onion. Finely grate or chop 2 garlic cloves.

2. Heat 1 tablespoon of the olive oil in a large Dutch oven or heavy-bottomed pot over medium-high heat until shimmering. Add 1 to 1 1/3 pounds lean ground beef and break it up with a wooden spoon. Let cook

undisturbed until the bottom is browned, about 5 minutes. Flip and continue to cook until cooked through and any liquid is evaporated, 2 to 3 minutes more.

3. Transfer the beef with a slotted spoon to a plate. Reduce the heat to medium. Add the remaining 2 tablespoons olive oil and onion. Cook, stirring occasionally and scraping any browned bits from the bottom, until the onions start to turn translucent, about 5 minutes. Meanwhile, bring 4 cups low-sodium beef broth to a boil in a medium saucepan over high heat. Add the celery and 1/2 teaspoon of the kosher salt and cook for 5 minutes. Drain the celery in a strainer set over a bowl; reserve the saucepan.

4. Add the celery, carrot, garlic, and 3 large fresh thyme sprigs to the onions. Cook, stirring occasionally, until the carrots start to slightly soften at the edges, about 5 minutes. Return the beef and any accumulated juices to the pot. While stirring continously, add 2 tablespoons tomato paste and sprinkle with 1/4 cup all-purpose flour. Cook, stirring often, until darkened in color, about 2 minutes.

5. Increase the heat to medium-high. Add 1 cup dry red wine and cook for 2 minutes to let alcohol to burn off.

Add the reserved broth and 1/4 cup Worcestershire sauce, and bring to a simmer.

6. Reduce the heat to low. Simmer uncovered, stirring occasionally, until the liquid thickens enough to coat the back of a spoon, about 45 minutes. Meanwhile, peel 2 1/2 pounds russet potatoes and cut into 1-inch pieces. Transfer to the reserved medium saucepan and add 2 bay leaves and enough cold water to cover the potatoes. Add 1 1/2 teaspoons of the kosher salt and 1/4 cup of the heavy cream if using. Bring to a boil over medium-high heat. Reduce teh heat as needed and simmer until the potatoes are tender, 15 to 20 minutes.

7. Meanwhile, arrange a rack in the upper third of the oven and heat the oven to 375°F. When the potatoes are almost ready, place 3/4 cup whole milk and 4 tablespoons unsalted butter in a small microwave-safe bowl. Microwave until the butter is melted and the milk is warm, 1 to 2 minutes. (Alternatively, heat in a small saucepan over medium-low heat.)

8. Drain the potatoes and discard the bay leaves. Return the potatoes to the pot. Place over low heat for 2 minutes, stirring regularly (this dries out potatoes and yields a fluffier mash). Remove the pot from the heat.

Pour in about half of the milk mixture and the remaining 1/4 cup heavy cream if using. Mash with a fork or potato masher until lightly mashed. Add the remaining milk mixture in 2 tablespoon increments, continuously beating with a fork, until smooth and creamy or the desired consistency is reached. Add the remaining 1 teaspoon kosher salt and 1/2 teaspoon ground white pepper or black pepper and stir to combine.

9. When the beef is ready, add the remaining 1 teaspoon kosher salt and 1/2 teaspoon ground white or black pepper, and stir to combine. Discard the thyme sprigs. Drain the ground beef mixture through a strainer set over a bowl (you should have about 2 cups gravy).

10. Transfer the beef mixture to an 8x8-inch baking dish and spread into an even layer. Spread the mashed potatoes evenly over the beef, completely covering it and going all the way to the edges of the baking dish. Use a fork to make lines, swirls, or patterns in the potatoes to create a crispy texture. Hold a box grater over the potatoes and grate 1 ounce aged cheddar or Parmesan cheese on the smallest holes evenly over the potatoes.

11. Bake until the cheese is melted and the topping is golden-brown in spots, 25 to 30 minutes. For an extra-crispy topping, turn the broiler on to high and broil until desired crispness, 3 to 5 minutes more. Let rest for 10 minutes before serving.

12. Rewarm the reserved gravy in the microwave for 1 to 2 minutes or in a small saucepan on the stovetop over medium heat for 2 to 3 minutes. Serve the cottage pie with a small drizzle of gravy on top.

30. Vegan Tacos with Smoky Chipotle Portobellos

Prep Time: 15 Minutes

Cook Time: 40 Minutes

Yield: serves8

Ingredients

- 2 extra large portobello mushrooms
- 1 red bell pepper
- ½ an onion – optional
- Chipotle Marindade
- 1 tablespoon oil
- 2 tablespoons canned Chipotle in Adobo sauce (SAUCE ONLY)
- 1 minced garlic clove (or ½ teaspoon granulated garlic)
- ½ teaspoon cumin
- ½ teaspoon coriander
- salt to taste
- 4 tortillas, warmed

- 1 can refried black beans, warmed
- Optional Garnishes: cilantro, pickled onions, Vegan Cilantro Crema or guacamole or sliced avocado.

Instructions

1. Preheat oven to 425F
2. Slice the portobellos into ½ inch thick wedges and slice bell pepper in to ½ thick strips. If adding onion, cut into ½ inch thick rings or half moons.
3. Place all on a sheet-pan lined sheet pan & Mix marinade ingredients together in a small bowl.
4. Brush both sides of mushrooms liberally with the marinade, then remaining red bell pepper and onion lightly. Sprinkle portobellos with salt. Roast 20 minutes or until portobellos are fork-tender.
5. While this is roasting, heat the beans any prep any additional garnishes. Pickled onions and Vegan cilantro Crema both take about 10 minutes to make. Or simply use avocado slices.
6. When ready to serve, warm the tortillas (over a gas flame on the stove, or in a toaster oven) and spread generously with the refried black beans. Divide chipotle portobellos and peppers (and onions if

used)among the tortillas. Top with Cilantro Crema, Poblano Salsa, or avocado, fresh cilantro and optional pickled onions.